Bed Yoga for Couples ~

Easy, Healing, Yoga Moves You Can Do in Bed

by

Blythe Ayne, Ph.D.

*Wedding ready, exercise
and mindfulness!

love
Gem
hehehe
xxx*

Bed Yoga for Couples ~

Easy, Healing, Yoga Moves You Can Do in Bed

by

Blythe Ayne, Ph.D.

Absolute Beginner Series – Book 3
Bed Yoga for Couples -
Easy, Healing, Yoga Moves You Can Do in Bed
Blythe Ayne, Ph.D.

Emerson & Tilman, Publishers
129 Pendleton Way #55
Washougal, WA 98671

Bed Yoga for Couples-
Easy, Healing, Yoga Moves You Can Do in Bed

ebook ISBN: 978-1-947151-73-4
Paperback ISBN: 978-1-947151-74-1
Hardbound ISBN: 978-1-947151-75-8
Large Print ISBN: 978-1-947151-76-5

[1. HEALTH & FITNESS/Yoga
2. HEALTH & FITNESS/Healing
3. BODY, MIND & SPIRIT/HEALING/Energy]

BIC: FM
First Edition

Thank you with deep appreciation
to all my brilliant & kind manuscript avatars.

DEDICATION:

With profound gratitude to all the awe-inspiring
Yoga instructors I've had through the years
And to yoga students everywhere.
Every day, we are *Absolute Beginners* –
Inspired by Anticipation, Serenity, and Joy.

Table of Contents

Bed Yoga for Couples

The Poses

Bed Yoga for Couples!

Fantastic! You're embarking on yoga for the two of you. There are so many wonderful advantages to doing yoga with a partner. You can each help the other stretch into the pose.

If it's a lazy Saturday morning and you don't feel like getting up just yet, you can ease into your day with a few shared yoga poses. It's a great way to feel connected, to hook up your energies and get on the same wavelength.

Or perhaps one of you is a bit under the weather. Your partner can help you get into a few gentle poses, which helps move your lymph about. This is an excellent way to stimulate healing and health.

Or one of you may be bedridden. Again, yoga is wonderful to not only move your lymph, but fire your muscles and work your joints. You and your partner may discover a perfect sequence of yoga movements that improves you, little by little.

Your lymph system is a network of tissues and organs that assist the body in clearing it of toxins and wastes. This system transports fluid lymph, which contains white blood cells, throughout your body, defending it against infections.

Unlike blood, which has the heart to pump it through your body, the lymph system is dependent on your movement to flow, and yoga is an excellent means to get it in motion!

As mentioned in my **Bed Yoga** book, going through yoga moves, even if only in your mind's eye, causes your muscles to fire. So let's get the lymph in motion and fire up some muscles!

The size and the firmness of your mattress will have a bearing on the *asanas* (Sanskrit for "pose"), as well as your own possible restrictions of movement. In the illustrations, the outline of a bed:

indicates a pose in a lying position.

Illustrations without the outline of a bed indicate the pose is seated or kneeling.

The most important point for the two of you to remember is that yoga is *about* you and *for* you. Although this book is laid out in a sequence of movements, you need only engage in the *asanas* that make you feel relaxed and strong.

Yoga is Not a Competition!

There's only happy, healthy, healing. Always communicate clearly with one another about any of the poses—if you'd like to go further into the movement, or if you've reached your "comfort zone."

Keep in mind that one of you is likely more flexible than the other, and one is possibly stronger. Both of those factors may be in the same partner, or one of you may be more flexible, while the other, stronger.

It's a fantastic opportunity to explore your wonderful differences, which includes being sensitive and responsive to the other's needs and limitations.

I love it that I never have to "be perfect" with yoga. I always get to be an *Absolute Beginner*—and so do you!

A Few Words About Format

Rather than refer to my enthusiastic stick people as "A" and "B," (which can be endlessly confusing!), I'll refer to their arms and legs as the "inside" or "outside" arms/legs, or, occasionally, "right" and "left" when both partners are using the same side.

So let's begin!

> Don't move the way fear makes you move~
> Move the way love makes you move.
> Osho

Shavasana

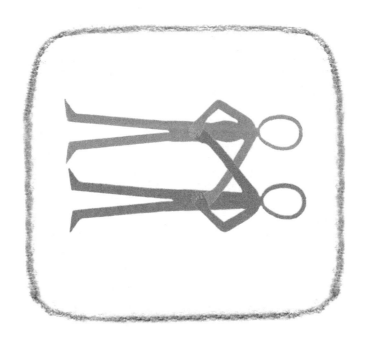

Movement:

Shavasana is a relaxed, meditative state of mind and body. You're both lying side-by-side, flat on your back with your arms at your sides and your feet relaxed a comfortable distance apart. What a great moment to engage with your partner in this relaxed, connected, state of being.

Let's set up a circuit of energy, from which your partner yoga will build a connection. Put your inside hand, face-up, on your partner's stomach, then hold their hand that's on your stomach with your other hand.

Feel your connected energy, a connected flow, and breath.

Breathe deeply—visualize oxygen being carried to every nook and cranny of your two bodies.

In this tranquil, calm, state of being, reflect on affirmations of love-sending and love-receiving, enjoying these meditative moments in calm repose.

You might picture your intentions for the day. See your day unfolding according to your heart's desire, meditatively, with equanimity, sailing through even moments of challenge.

This is your private connection between you and your partner. You may reflect in meditative quiet, or you might share an affirmation, an insight, a blessing.

You may discover that you're quite moved by this energy flow. Relax into it. Nurture the healing, cherish the moment.

Whether your affirmations or insights are shared or quietly reflected upon, remain mindful of your breathing. Breath deeply, inhaling and exhaling—feel your stomach rising and falling. Feel your partner's stomach rising and falling. Feel the rhythm of life, releasing it all into the breath.

It's good to be mindful of total, deep, breathing.

Let everything go, relaxing. *Relax.*

There is nothing to worry about. There's nothing to do. Feel your mind relaxing. Your face relaxes. Your arms and your hands ... relax. Your chest and your abdomen ... relax. Your legs and your feet ... relax. *You completely ... relax....*

> When the breath is calmed
> the mind will be still.
> Hatha Yoga Pradipika

Side Bend (reclined) – Urdhva Hastasana

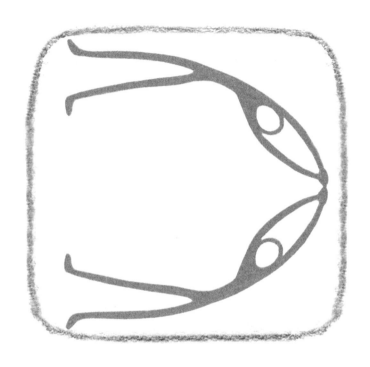

Movement:

When you're ready to move, reach your hands overhead. Stretch toward one another. Crossing your wrists, hold your partner's hands, and gently pull into a full extension of your body—feel this stretch from your fingers to your toes.

Hold this position for several breaths. Breathe deeply, mindfully sensing the life-giving breath nurturing your ribs, your spinal cord, your brain, and your organs.

After several breaths, release your handhold and stretch away from each other. Intertwine your fingers and give yourself a nice, full, fingers-to-toes stretch for an equal amount of time.

Benefits:
Side bends activate your core muscles, expand your ribs, and deepen your breath, stimulating the flow of blood and energy through your organs and improving circulation.

The movement increases the range of motion and elasticity of your spine, which in turn feeds your brain, augmenting the flow of cerebrospinal fluid.

Keeps you youthful and flexible!

> Meditation is a way
> For nourishing and blossoming
> The divinity within you.
> Amit Ray

Reclining Spinal Twist – Jathara Parivartanasana

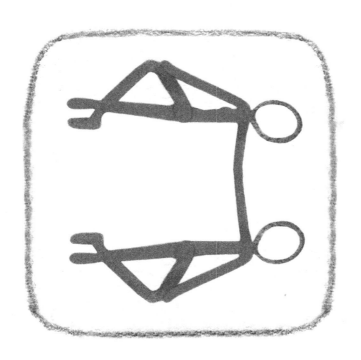

Movement:

Begin by lying side by side on your back with a bit of space between you, hugging your knees to your chest. Then slowly extend your outside leg.

Guide your bent knee across your body with the opposite hand, away from your partner. Gently relax your knee to the bed.

Extend your inner arm toward your partner. Holding one another's extended forearm, turn your head toward your partner. Engage a gentle isometric pull from one hand to the other, while keeping both shoulders touching the bed.

Inhale energy, exhale tension, moving more deeply into the pose.

Feel your spine relax. Gradually let your shoulders melt in relaxation. Feel your bent knee gently giving in to the reclining twist.

After relaxing into the twist for several breaths, return to hugging your knees.

Then slowly extend your inner leg, guiding the outside bent knee across your body toward your partner. Extend your outside arm, and turn your head toward the extended arm, away from your partner, keeping your shoulders touching the bed.

Inhale energy, exhale tension, moving more deeply into the pose.

Feel your spine relaxing, let your shoulders melt in relaxation as your bent knee gently gives in to the reclining twist.

Hold the pose for several breaths.

Benefits:

Twists help wring out toxins in your organs—and along with the toxins, the anxious and exhausted emotions that often accompany these toxins melt away.

Reclining Spinal Twist stimulates the flow of fresh blood to digestive organs and strengthens abdominal muscles. It stretches your back muscles and glutes, and gives your back and hips a healthy massage.

Twists also hydrate, lengthen, relax, and realign your spine.

A gentle spinal twist first thing in the morning, or in the evening after a taxing day, provides body-wide healing.

> Yoga is the fountain of youth.
> Bob Harper

Reclining Triangle – Utthita Trikonasana

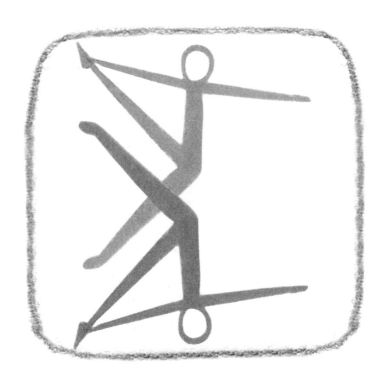

Movement:

Several of the poses in *Bed Yoga for Couples* are adapted from standing poses into reclining poses. Practicing standing poses in a reclined position is an excellent way to become familiar with the form of a pose.

The first standing pose we'll practice in a reclined position is *Reclining Triangle*. Lie side by side. Move your feet wide apart with your inside leg crossing your partner's leg. Turn your outside foot flat against the bed while keeping the inside foot pointing up. With your legs extended, lift your knee caps and keep your knees in line with your big toes.

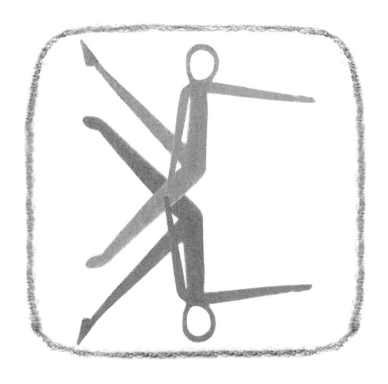

Bend over at the waist, away from your partner. Stretch your arms out in a straight line, one hand touching your foot and the other overhead, extending energetically through to the ends of your fingertips. Then both partners reach the bottom hand—the one touching your foot—toward each other and hold hand-to-wrist. Exert a gentle isometric pull, which you extend throughout your body.

Inhaling deeply, lengthen through your ribs. Keep your neck in line with your spine, looking down at your foot, or up at your extended hand, whichever is comfortable.

Relax into the pose, breathing deeply. When you're ready to move to the other side, release your handhold and orient your feet in the opposite positions, then repeat the pose on the other side.

Throughout the pose, keep your legs engaged, lengthening through your ribs, your arms, and the crown of your head.

Benefits:
What's great about doing a standing pose in a reclined position is that if and when you take a standing pose to the mat, you've become familiar with how your body feels when in perfect alignment, as you're in perfect alignment with your back against the bed. The pose will be beautiful and beneficial, both reclining and standing.

Triangle pose stretches your thighs, hamstrings, calves, shoulders, chest, and spine, and is great for making your hips more flexible. It can also be helpful with sciatica. It stimulates your organs which improves metabolism.

Trikonasana improves both physical and mental balance and stability, and is known to be therapeutic for anxiety.

> Yoga adds years to your life
> And life to your years.
> Alan Finger

Staff Pose – Dandasana

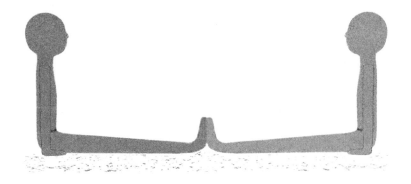

Movement:

Staff pose is an active-without-movement pose. Sit facing one another with your legs together and outstretched. Keep your back perfectly straight with your hands on the bed, facing forward next to your hips.

Flex your feet, pushing through your heels into your partner's heels while actively pressing your sitting bones into the bed. Draw your abdomen in and up to help you sit straight.

Draw your shoulders down and toward each other, opening your chest. Be sure your shoulders are over your hips. Tuck your chin slightly, picturing your neck long and your ears in line with your shoulders.

Breathe deeply in this pose for several breaths with the abdominal muscles engaged, remaining active-yet-relaxed in the pose.

Benefits:

Staff Pose improves core stability and strengthens your back muscles and your quads.

It improves your posture, and sets you up for the next upward-facing poses.

> Contemplate that which is sublime ~
> In this way, you become sublime.
> Blythe Ayne

Seated Forward Bend – Paschimottanasana

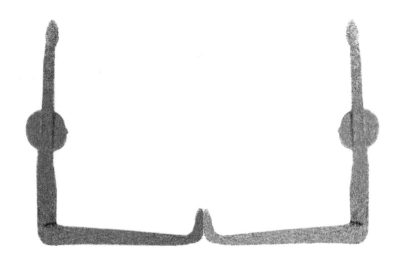

Movement:
Sit facing each other with your legs outstretched and your feet flexed. Inhale and lengthen your spine, then raise your arms straight overhead, alongside your ears.

Picture the front of your body open and long. Exhale and gently begin to fold forward, hinging from your hips, keeping the spine straight. Feel the movement in your chest, ribcage, and stomach as you move your forehead toward your legs.

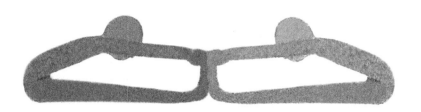

Reach your hands to the bottoms of your feet. If you can't reach your feet, bend your knees slightly until you can wrap your index finger and thumb around your big toes. Continue to gently extend your legs. Reach your partner's toes if you can.

Inhale and exhale slowly and mindfully, concentrating on hinging at your hips. Keep your arms lifted, pull your shoulders away from your ears, while keeping your collar bones wide.

On the in-breath, lengthen the front of your torso. On the out-breath, fold deeper into the bend, hinging from the hips with a straight spine, while keeping your neck in line with your spine.

Breathe into your *Seated Forward Bend* as long as it feels good.

Benefits:
The benefits of a relaxing-yet-mindful *Seated Forward Bend* are plentiful. It stretches the spine, shoulders, and hamstrings.

It stimulates the organs and aids digestion.

It is therapeutic for insomnia, sinusitis, high blood pressure, and depression.

Relax into a calm *Seated Forward Bend* any time stressors threaten to overwhelm you.

> Yoga is the process of eliminating pain ~
> Pain from the body, mind, and society.
> Amit Ray

Boat Pose – Paripurna Navasana

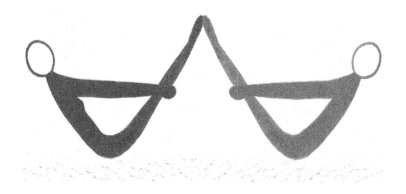

Movement:

Begin in a sitting position facing one another. Bend your knees with your feet on the bed. Place your hands slightly behind your hips, fingers facing forward.

Lengthen your spine, open your collar bones wide to open the chest while drawing in your abdominal muscles.

Both you and your partner lean back on your sitting bones and lift your feet, with the bottoms of your feet touching.

Keep your spine straight and your chest open, then extend your arms parallel to the bed. Picture your thigh bones, attached to your hip flexors, as anchors to the bottom of your spine, from which your spine and your thighs raise in a strong "V." Breath deeply into the pose.

Hold one another's wrists if you both can reach.

At first, you may not be able to raise your calves into a 45-degree angle. That will come with practice. What's important is to keep your spine and thighs in the 45-degree angle, while bending at the knees.

If you have lower back pain, move into boat pose gently. Though it will strengthen your lower back over time, do not engage in it to the point of pain.

Benefits:
Boat pose stimulates digestion and improves core strength.

But most importantly, it strengthens your hip flexors that attach your inner thigh bones to the front of your spine.

Boat pose is also known for relieving stress.

> Yoga is a light which once lit will never dim
> The better your practice
> The brighter your flame
> B.K.S. Iyengar

Seated Side Angle Bend – Parsva Upavistha Konasana

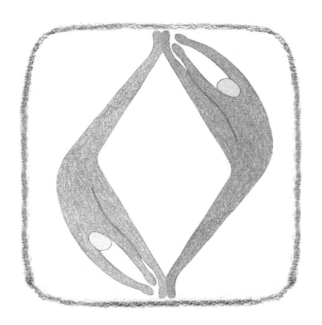

Movement:

Face one another in *Staff Pose*, keeping your spines long, and legs straight out in front. Then move your legs into as wide an angle as you comfortably can, while keeping the integrity of your straight spine.

Touching the bottoms of your feet with your partner's, flex your feet, keeping your knees and toes pointed up. Press your legs and sitting bones down while lengthening through your spine, tilting your pubic bone up and back to assist in keeping the spine straight.

Both partners twist from the waist to face your right legs. As you exhale, walk your hands toward your right foot, while reaching your forehead toward your knee. The goal is to hold onto your right foot, but if you're not there yet, hold onto your shin or ankle. When you reach your pose, relax your elbows, shoulders, and neck.

If you have reached your foot, you can deepen the pose by reaching for your partner's toes. Hold for several breaths, relaxing into the pose.

Alternately, you can hold each other's left wrist while still reaching for your right toes, adding a bit of isometric to the pose.

Release the pose by slowly walking your hands back to your waist and gently rolling up your spine returning to your seated staff pose. Then repeat the movements on your left side.

Benefits:
Seated Side Angle Bend opens and stretches your hips and the backs of your legs, while strengthening your spine. It stimulates the abdominal organs and provides deep relaxation.

Bend so you don't break.
Unknown

Wide-Angle Seated Forward Fold – Paschimottanasana

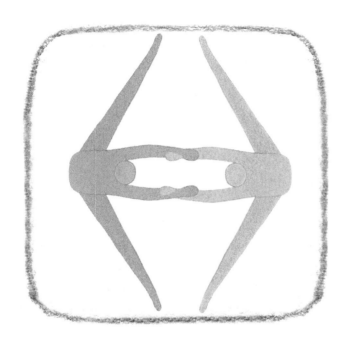

Movement:

Facing one another in *Staff Pose*, sit with your spine long, and your legs straight out in front. Then move your legs into as wide an angle as you comfortably can, while keeping the integrity of your straight spine, touching the bottoms of your feet with your partner's.

Flex your feet, keeping your knees and toes pointed up. Press your legs and sitting bones down while lengthening through your spine, tilting your pubic bone up and back to assist in keeping the spine straight. Begin to bend from your hips, not your back, and place your hands in front of you on the bed. Slowly exhale, pushing your hands forward.

When you and your partner's hands meet, hold one another's wrists. Keep the front of your body long and straight as you come forward, lengthening from pubic bone to breast bone. When you feel your back begin to arch, pause, breathing deeply. On an exhalation, move deeper into the pose if you can. When you reach your limit of stretching your hands forward while keeping your back straight, you will feel the stretch along the back of your legs.

Stay in this pose for several breaths, feeling the energy of the stretch in your legs. Then return to your seated position, coming up with a straight back, while pressing your sitting bones down.

Benefits:
Wide-Angle Seated Forward Fold opens and stretches the entire back of your body, your hips, and the inside of your legs, while strengthening your spine. It has

the wonderful attribute of stimulating the abdominal organs while providing deep relaxation.

> If your compassion
> Does not include yourself
> It is incomplete.
> Jack Kornfield

Garland Pose (Squat) – Malasana

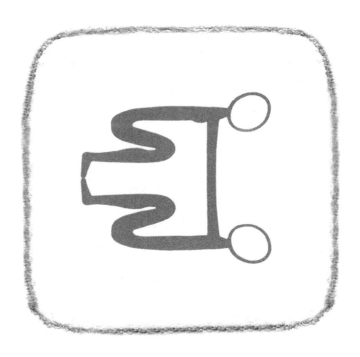

Movement:

Let's become familiar with *Garland Pose* by practicing it lying on the bed, though it is generally done from a standing position. A full squat is challenging for people with limited flexibility, but a bit of practice in a side-lying position will be helpful with the poses engaging *Garland* further along in this book.

Lie facing each other and hold onto one another's wrists. Both partners slowly bend both knees until the pelvis is resting at the back of the heels. If you cannot do this at first, be patient. You'll be pleased to discover that gradually, as you continue to practice *Garland Pose*, your knees become stronger and more flexible.

Benefits:
The benefits of *Malasana* are numerous! It contributes to flexible knees, strengthens hamstrings, gluteal muscles, calf muscles, and lower back.

It aids digestion by stimulating the digestive organs, and it tones the belly muscles.

> Yoga shines the light of awareness
> Into the darkest corners of the body.
> Jason Crandell

Low Lunge – Ashwa Sanchalasana

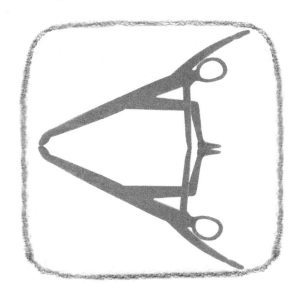

Movement:

Facing each other in your side-lying position, both partners slide their bottom leg into a bent knee position, bottoms of feet touching.

Your top legs are straight, with the tips of the toes touching.

Raise your bottom arm overhead—your bodies are now in a straight line from fingertips to toes.

With your top arm, hold onto each other's wrist and pull gently for several deep breaths, maintaining the beautiful straight line of your bodies.

Relax from the pose by releasing the wrist-hold and straightening the bent knee.

Then repeat the sequence on the opposite side.

Benefits:
Low lunge strengthens and stretches legs, knees and ankles, helps alleviate low back pain, and stimulates the abdominal organs.

It contributes to building mental focus and concentration, while calming the mind.

> Yoga is not about self~improvement
> It's about self~acceptance.
> Gurmukh Kaur Khalsa

Reclined Forward Bend —Uttanasana

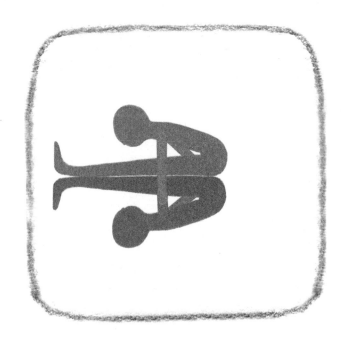

Movement:

Lying back to back, both partners bend forward, reaching for your toes. Lie your bottom arm alongside your torso or overhead, whichever is more comfortable.

When you have reached your comfortable forward bend, reach back with your top arm and hold your partner's wrist, then gently pull further into the bend. Do not force it or go farther than is comfortable! As always, each partner must honor the other's limits.

You'll discover that, over time, you'll be able to go farther and deeper into your reclining forward bend.

Benefits:
Forward Bend stretches your hips, hamstrings, and calves, strengthens your knees, while massaging your internal organs.

It relieves stress, depression, and anxiety while quieting the mind.

> Center your body and mind
> Stretch the possibilities.
> Unknown

Camel Pose – Ustrasana

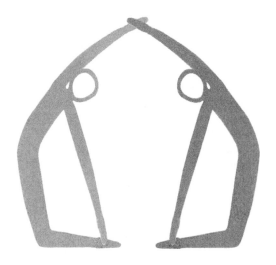

Movement:

Begin by kneeling on the bed back to back, with a few inches distance from your partner's feet. Align your knees with your hips, and keep your shins parallel.

Place your hands on your lower back, fingers pointing down, guiding the tailbone down. Inhale, bringing your shoulder blades down toward your ribs, and lift your heart.

Lean back, but do not drop your head. Both partners raise the outer arm and reach to hold hands. With your other arm, you can either reach for your foot, or simply leave the hand on your lower back.

If raising the arm up and back is uncomfortable at first, keep both hands on the lower back.

Remain here for several deep breaths, then switch arms.

Relax from this position by sitting your hips on your heels for a few breaths.

Benefits:
Camel Pose stretches the neck, chest, abdomen, hip flexors and thighs, while strengthening the back and glutes, and it will enhance your posture.

It stimulates the energy centers in your body.

> Yoga doesn't take time
> It gives time.
> Ganga White

Child's Pose – Balasana

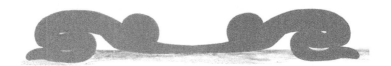

Movement:

Both partners kneel on the bed facing one another, with enough distance between you to reach forward with your arms.

Your knees are a bit wider than your hips, with toes touching.

Extend your arms in front and hold onto your partner's forearms with a gentle pull.

Exhaling, relax your stomach between your thighs, while pulling back onto your heels, or as close to them as you can. For more, you can raise your elbows off the bed. Or to fully relax in the pose, let your elbows rest on the bed.

Rest your forehead on the bed. If your head does not easily rest on the bed, use pillows under your head until you can rest comfortably. Stay in this resting pose for as long as it feels good. Either partner may return to *Child's Pose* at any time if needing a few moments to relax and recharge.

Benefits:
Along with being an excellent few moments of relaxation, *Child's Pose* gently stretches your shoulders, lower back, hips, thighs, ankles, and knees.

It helps to relieve fatigue, increases blood circulation to your head, and calms your mind and body.

> Yoga is the exploration and discovery
> Of the subtle energies of life.
> Amit Ray

Dolphin –
Ardha Pincha Mayurasnana

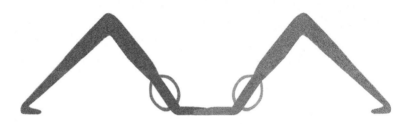

Movement:

If you are moving into *Dolphin*, from *Child's Pose*, both partners leave their arms in extended embrace, elbows on the bed.

Then raise your hips up into a pointed, upside-down "V." Open your shoulders wide, and inhale deeply. Keep your knees slightly bent, with more attention given to keeping your spine long and straight.

Gradually straighten your legs and reach your heels toward the bed. Continue to picture your spine straight, while drawing the muscles of your legs in and up.

Extend your hips upward, and pull your shoulder blades down, maintaining the width between them. Keep your neck relaxed, aligned with your spine, and align your head with your arms.

Hold this position for several deep breaths, visualizing your spine straight, with each vertebra and disk being nurtured by the reverse flow of blood and spinal fluid in the space between them.

Benefits:
This is an excellent alternate pose for *Downward Dog*. *Dolphin* strengthens and stretches your shoulders, arms, and legs, and is great for the arches of your feet.

It improves digestion and calms the mind, while helping to relieve stress and depression.

> Watch that which watches ~
> Attune to the third eye.
> Blythe Ayne

Child's Pose – Balasana
& Fish Pose – Matsyasana

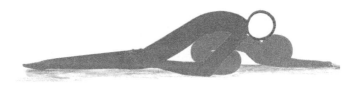

Movement:
Let's move into poses where each partner engages in a different pose.

One partner relaxes into *Child's Pose*, as previously described.

The other partner begins *Fish Pose* by first lying back to back on the partner in *Child's Pose*. Place your hands on the tops of your thighs, and, with toes flexed or extended, keep your feet and your toes engaged.

Inhale deeply while pressing your elbows down toward the bed. The support of the partner in *Child's Pose* automatically lifts your chest, which is the essence of *Fish Pose*. Pull your shoulders together and move to rest the top of your head between your partner's shoulders.

Relax into this pose for several deep breaths. Then switch poses.

Benefits:

The benefits of *Child's Pose* are as mentioned, above. In addition, the weight of your partner along your back helps you engage more fully in a heel-reaching *Child's Pose*.

Fish Pose stretches the intercostal muscles between the ribs, opens the chest, and opens and stimulates the throat.

It also has an amazing ability to relieve irritation and that "grindy" feeling one gets from over-stimulation, frustration, and, simply, those "bad traffic" days.

> Expect nothing
> Appreciate everything.
> Unknown

Bow – Dhanurasana

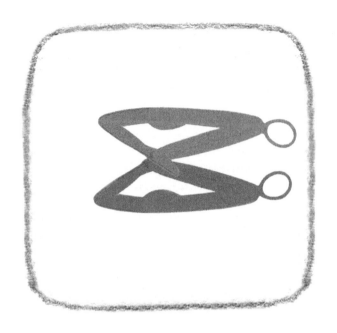

Movement:

You both lie on your side, back to back, with enough space between you to reach back and grab your feet.

Exhale, bending your knees as much as you can and grab your ankles. Pull your navel toward your spine, and push your ankles into your hands, arching gently through your back, with head and chin slightly tucked. Keeping the back of your neck long. Press your shoulder blades back to open your heart.

You can then reach for your partner's feet. One partner may be able to reach the partner's feet, while the other may not yet be able to reach his or her own feet. For either or both partners who have reached the other's feet, pull gently, to allow a deeper engagement with bow, but *be very gentle* with this back-arching pose.

Breathe deeply into your back for several breaths before releasing with control. Then roll onto your stomach, make a pillow with your forearms and relax fully, inhaling and exhaling deeply.

Benefits:
Bow pose strengthens your back, opens your chest, and stretches the front of your body.

It energizes your whole body, stimulates your organs, and eases anxiety.

> Yoga is not about touching your toes,
> It's what you learn on the way there.
> Jigar Gor

Pigeon –
Utthita Eka Pada Kapotasana

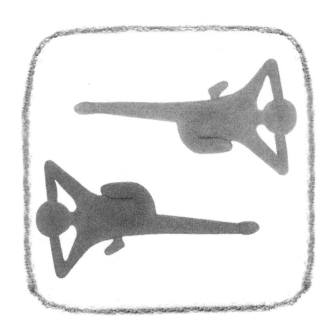

Movement:

Lying on your stomach, come up on all fours, hands under shoulders and knees under hips.

Bring your right knee forward and place it behind your right wrist, with your ankle in front of your left hip. Try to get your shin in a straight line behind your two hands, though this may be difficult at first.

Slide your left leg straight behind you, making sure that it's not drawing out to the side. Straighten your left knee and point your toes. Keep the right foot flexed.

Gently lower your torso over your bent leg. Keep your hips level with one another—the tendency is for the crossed leg to lower that hip. Place a pillow or folded blanket under your right hip if it is difficult to get your hips to stay level.

Be mindful of your bent knee. If this pose troubles your knees, you can do it lying on your back, extending your left leg on the bed and holding your right bent leg across your torso with your hands.

Breathing deeply, stay in *Pigeon* for several breaths, continuing to release the tension in the right hip.

To come out of the pose, push yourself up with your hands and return to all fours. Then repeat the movement on the other side.

Although there is no partner interaction in this pose, you can take turns assisting one another in gently bringing the knee forward and getting the shin in a straight line and keeping the hips level. *Offer any assistance gently!*

Benefits:

Pigeon opens your hips, using core strength to keep your hips level, while stretching your thighs, psoas (the large muscles that run from the lumbar spine and through the groin that flex the hip) and groin. When you can fully relax into *Pigeon* it is wonderfully calming.

> More stretching
> Less stressing.
> Unknown

Back to Back Meditation/Easy Pose – *Sukhasana*

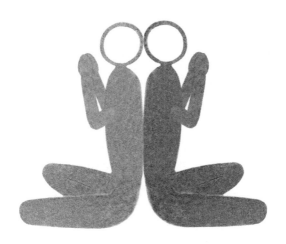

Movement:

Sit back to back. Straighten you back against your partner's back for mutual support. You might want to sit on a folded blanket to keep your hips in line with, or a bit above, your knees. Cross your legs in a comfortable position.

Continue to straighten and lengthen your spine, creating length through your spine to the crown of your head. Firm your shoulder blades.

There are a variety of hand positions. You can hold them, palms together, at your heart chakra to create a heart-centered circuit. Or you may place your hands on your knees. Place your palms down for a calming effect, or facing up for an energizing effect.

Relax in this meditative position for a few minutes. You can also, during your meditation, cross your legs the opposite way. Although this will likely feel awkward, it's good for both your brain and your physical flexibility.

One partner may become engaged in a personal meditation for a longer period, during which time the other partner may practice one of the other asanas.

Benefits:
Easy Pose or *Happy Sitting Pose* as it's also called, strengthens your back, and opens your hips.

It calms your mind, and is good for preparing you to do breathing exercises or to allow for a centering meditation.

> Let your yoga practice
> Be a celebration of life.
> Seido lee de Barros

Easy Seated Twist –
Parivrtta Sukhasana

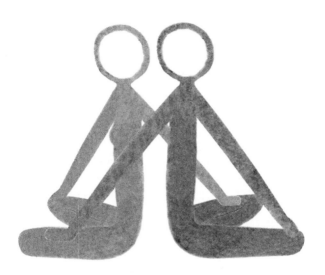

Movement:

Both partners sit back to back in a comfortable, cross-legged position. Then both partners raise your right arm and twist to place your right hand on your own left knee, palm down.

Next, reach your left arm out to the left and place your left hand, palm down, on your partner's right thigh or knee.

Breathe deeply and continue to gently twist to your left as far as you can for several breaths.

Then relax from the position for two or three breaths and repeat the twist the other direction, raising your left arm and twisting to place your left hand on your own right knee, palm down.

Then reach the right arm to the right and place your right hand, palm down, on your partner's left thigh or knee.

Breathe deeply and continue to gently twist to your right as far as you can for several breaths.

Benefits:
Easy Seated Twist helps your spine maintain, and even *increase*, its range of motion.

It relieves backache and sciatica.

It provides an excellent stretch for your hips, shoulders, and neck, while squeezing toxins out of your organs and improving your digestion.

It reduces stress and anxiety and boosts your energy.

> You are one yoga workout
> Away from a good mood.
> Unknown

Easy Pose with Cactus Arms – *Sukhasana*

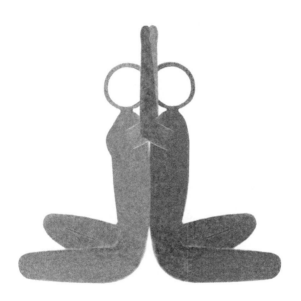

Movement:

Sit back to back in a comfortable, cross-legged position and raise your arms to a 90-degree position, your palms back to back with your partner's palms.

Squeeze your shoulder blades together, opening your chest. Intertwine your forearms with your partner's so your palms are facing. Push gently for an isometric engagement. If your palms do not come face to face, or if you're not flexible enough yet to intertwine your forearms, engage in the pose to your comfort, and, as always, be mindful of the needs of your partner.

Hold the pose for several deep breaths.

Benefits:
Easy Pose with Cactus Arms strengthens your upper back and shoulders, while opening the heart center, which contributes to a better connection between the two of you.

> The mind lives in doubt
> The heart lives in trust ~
> When you trust
> You become centered.
> Osho

A few Words About Inversions

Inversions lower high blood pressure and improve blood circulation, which provides more oxygen and blood to the brain, augmenting memory, concentration, and mental processing. Just 3 to 5 minutes of inversion allows the tired blood of your lower limbs to flow rapidly back to the heart, where it refreshes.

In an inversion, tissue fluids can flow more efficiently into the veins and lymph system of your lower limbs and abdominal and pelvic organs, providing a healthy exchange of nutrients and wastes between cells and capillaries.

Legs Up the Wall – Viparita Karani

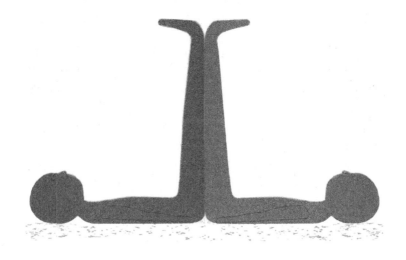

Movement:

Legs up the Wall is a great inversion! Both partners lie on your side with your legs back to back, while bending away from each other at the waist in a 90-degree angle.

Then lift your legs straight up in the air, resting your legs against your partner's legs.

Relax your arms at your sides, palms facing up. Using one another as a wall, relax your feet, your calves, your thighs, relax your abdomen, your chest, your head, your arms, and hands—just r-e-l-a-x.

Breathing deeply, remain in the pose for several deep breaths, or even several minutes if you feel inclined, enjoying the relaxation and rejuvenation.

To come out of the pose, gently slide your legs down opposite your partner and use your hands to come to a seated position.

You can also use the wall at the head of your bed for individual *Legs Up the Wall*. Here, too, you can help one another get into the pose.

Benefits:

Legs Up the Wall has numerous benefits for mind, body, and spirit. Ancient texts say this pose will destroy old age. It stretches the back of your legs, and relieves cramps in legs and feet. It reduces swollen ankles and calves, and stretches your torso and the back of your neck.

Legs up the Wall relieves anxiety, headaches, migraine, backaches, insomnia, mild depression, muscle fatigue, arthritis, both high and low blood pressure, varicose veins, and cramps.

It strengthens your immune system, balances your hormonal system, calms your nervous system, stabilizes your digestive and elimination systems, and regulates your respiratory system.

Not bad for a nice, relaxing asana!

> Sky above
> Earth below
> Peace within.
> Unknown

Garland Pose – Malasana &
Legs Up the Wall – Viparita Karani

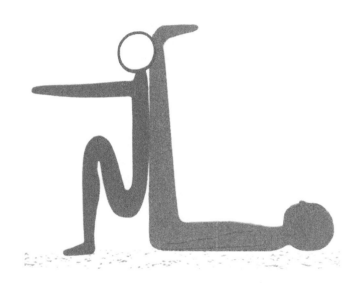

Movement:
Let's engage two poses that we've already explored. One partner moves into *Legs Up the Wall* – without the wall.

The other partner leans against the first partner's legs and moves down into *Garland Pose*. Maintain this pose for several breaths.

After coming out of these poses, you reverse positions.

Benefits:
The benefits of these two poses in conjunction with one another offer all the benefits of each as already

stated. In addition, they provide an opportunity for you to explore your edge, with the new combination of muscles and different forms of support.

> Yoga poses are useful maps to explore yourself
> But they are not the territory.
> Donna Farhi

Bridge Pose – Setu Bandhasana & Garland Pose – Malasana

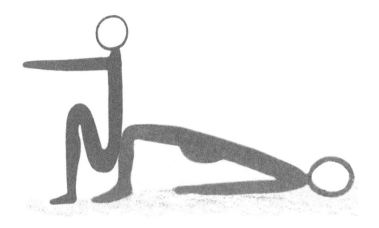

Movement:

Another two-pose movement is *Garland Pose* and *Bridge Pose*.

The first partner moves into *Bridge Pose* by lying on your back with knees bent. The soles of your feet are on the bed, with your knees pointing to the ceiling. Your feet are parallel to each other, your heels are right under your knees.

Place your arms along your sides, palms facing down. On your exhale, press your feet firmly into the bed, and lift your tailbone, then your lower back, and then your mid-back, while pressing your knees forward.

Lift your chest. Keep your thighs parallel.

While the first partner holds *Bridge Pose*, the other partner moves into *Garland Pose*, using the knees of the partner in *Bridge Pose* as support.

Hold this pose for a few breaths, then both partners relax for a few breaths before changing positions and repeating the sequence.

Benefits:
The benefits of *Garland Pose* are as previously stated—contributing to flexible knees, strengthened hamstrings, gluteal muscles, calf muscles, and lower back, and aiding digestion.

Bridge Pose is a great stretch for your chest, neck, and spine.

It improves digestion and reduces insomnia.

It's also a great moment to contemplate any bridges you may be crossing in life. Perhaps your yoga *Bridge Pose* will help clarify where you intend to be when you cross your life bridge.

> Yoga exists in the world
> Because everything is linked.
> Desikasha

Warrior Poses

Let's take the *Warrior Poses* to the bed! As previously mentioned, the advantage of practicing standing poses while lying down is that, although they're not the same as when weight-bearing, you'll get the *feel* of your body in proper alignment. This can be a significant advantage when you take these poses to the mat.

Warrior I Pose – Verabhadrasana I

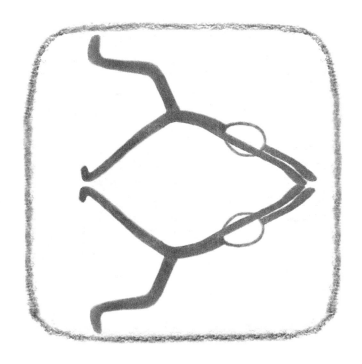

Movement:

Lying back to back, move down on the bed far enough to be able to raise your arms overhead.

Both partners stretch your legs into a wide "V," then bend the outside knee to a 90-degree angle. Turn your inside foot so your toes point to the ceiling, while your outside foot is lying flat on the bed.

Make sure that your hips are in line with one another, and keep your torso in a straight line over your hips. Engage your leg muscles.

Inhale and lift your arms overhead, pulling your shoulders down away from your ears. Elongate your spine, open your collarbones, and lift your breastbone. Firm your triceps to raise your arms further.

You can hold hands overhead if you easily reach one another.

Hold the pose for ten or fifteen slow breaths, or longer if it feels beneficial, then relax onto your back, bringing your feet together and your arms to your sides. Then switch places to repeat the movements on your opposite side.

Benefits:
Warrior I opens your hip joints and helps to alleviate painful conditions involving the sacrum. It improves posture and stretches your ankles, calves, and thighs.

It improves the mobility in your shoulders, while opening your chest and lungs.

All the warrior poses augment your mind-body connection, opening the heart to stimulate emotional strength. They also support the parasympathetic nervous system, which in turn sustains equanimity.

> Yoga provides an inner quiet
> Where you can release the outer noisy.
> Blythe Ayne

Humble Warrior –
Baddha Verabhadrasana

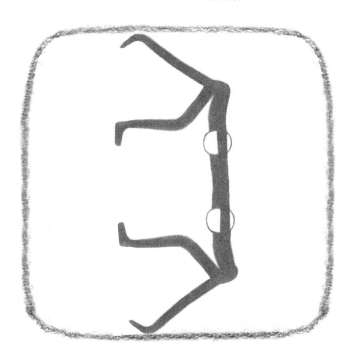

Movement:
Lying face to face, both partners stretch your legs into a wide "V." Then you both bend the inside knee to a 90-degree angle.

Make sure to keep your hips in alignment while keeping your torso squarely over your hips. Engage your leg muscles.

Reach your arms forward and hold each other's forearms, bending and extending your torso toward your knee.

Keep your legs, arms, and torso engaged and bring your torso toward your front bent knee, with your chest coming into contact with your thigh if possible.

After several energizing breaths, relax from the pose. Then reverse the positions of the legs and repeat the pose with the other leg.

Benefits:
Humble Warrior opens your lungs and chest and stretches your arms, legs, back, and neck. It is a deep hip opener.

It stimulates the nervous system and the abdominal organs, encouraging feelings of quiet strength while inspiring equanimity and acceptance.

> Yoga means union ~
> The union of body with consciousness
> And consciousness with the soul.
> B.K.S. Iyengar

Warrior II Pose – Verabhadrasana II

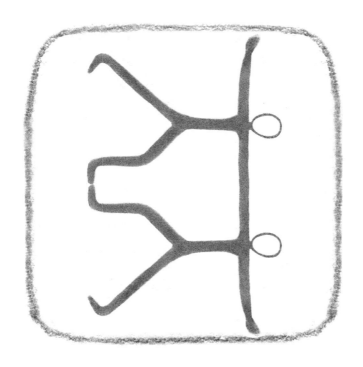

Movement:

You both lie flat on your back. Move your legs to a wide-legged stance, and, on an inhale, raise your arms in a straight line to shoulder level, keeping your shoulders down and your neck long. Exhale and bend your inside knee until it is in line with your ankle.

Engage your hips and elongate through the length of your spine. Draw your abdomen in and up while keeping your diaphragm soft. Extend from your collarbones out through the tips of your fingers. Draw your tailbone toward your feet to lengthen your lower back. Be sure your shoulders are in line with your hips.

Fix your gaze beyond your inside fingertips toward your partner, imagining a bright and calm future.

Remain in this meditative pose for as long as it feels energizing. Relax from the pose by returning your arms to your sides and your legs extended straight, then repeat the sequence on the other side, exhaling and bending your outside knee until it is in line with your ankle, with your gaze facing away from your partner.

Benefits:
Warrior II opens your hips and stretches your thighs, chest, lungs, and shoulders, and increases stamina.

It also opens your heart to wisdom, and steadies your intention, bringing a centered power to your daily life.

> The heart of yoga is a steady effort
> In the direction you want to go.
> Sally Kempton

Reverse Warrior Pose – Viparita Verabhadrasana

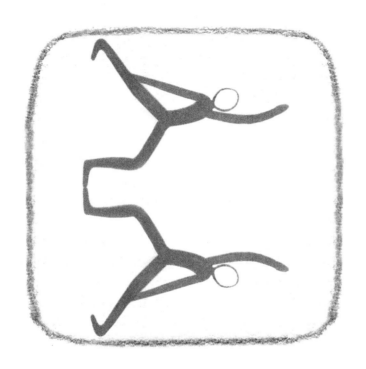

Movement:

Reverse Warrior starts in a *Warrior II* stance. You both lie flat on your back and move your legs apart to a wide-legged stance. On an inhale, raise your arms to shoulder level, keeping your shoulders down and your neck long. Exhale and bend your inside knee until it is in line with your ankle.

Engage your hips and elongate through the length of your spine. Draw your abdomen in and up, while keeping your diaphragm soft. Extend from your collarbones out through the tips of your fingers. Draw your tailbone toward your feet to lengthen your lower back. Be sure that your shoulders are in line with your hips.

Inhaling, turn the palm of your inside hand up, extending your arm overhead, while sliding your other arm down your straight leg toward the back of your knee.

Firm your shoulder blades, lift your chest and move into a gentle backbend. Raise your head and gaze at your right hand breathing deeply for several breaths.

Gently relax, then repeat the movements on your opposite side.

Benefits:
Reverse Warrior opens your chest, side body, hips, groin, and legs. It improves flexibility of the spine, and releases tension in the intercostal muscles around your ribs, while encourages deeper breathing.

It's relaxing while at the same time, energizing, and is known to improve self-esteem.

> Being present changes you.
> Mariel Hemingway

Excellent!

You've worked your way through **Bed Yoga for Couples**—*congratulations!* Now is a good time to return to *Shavasana*, to let the two of you become completely relaxed, while body, mind, and spirit integrate the beneficial work you've done. Peacefully-yet-mindfully let every cell of your bodies heal and rejuvenate.

Shavasana

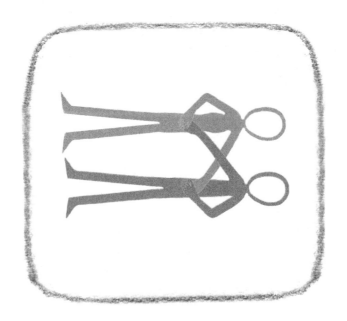

Movement:

We come now, full circle, to *Shavasana*—the completely relaxed, meditative state of mind and body.

You're both lying flat on your back with your arms at your sides and your feet relaxed a comfortable distance apart. What a great moment to engage with your partner in this relaxed, connected, state of being.

Let's return to that circuit of energy. Put your inside hand, face-up, on your partner's stomach. Then hold their hand that's on your stomach with your other hand. Feel the connected energy and the breath.

Breathe deeply—visualize oxygen being carried to every nook and cranny of your two bodies.

In this tranquil, calm, state of being, reflect on affirmations of love-sending and love-receiving. Enjoy these meditative moments in calm repose.

Move through your day in your mind's eye, meditatively, with equanimity, sailing through even moments of challenge.

This is your very private space between you and your partner. You may reflect in meditative quiet, or you may share an affirmation, an insight, or a blessing.

You may discover that you're quite moved by this energy flow. Relax into it. Nurture the healing, cherish the moment.

Whether your affirmations or insights are shared or quietly reflected upon, remain mindful of your breathing. Breath deeply, inhaling and exhaling—feel your stomach rising and falling. Feel your partner's stomach rising and falling. Feel the rhythm of life and love.

Then release it all into the breath.

It's good to be mindful of total, deep, breathing.

Let everything go, relaxing. *Relax.*

There is nothing to worry about. There's nothing to do.
Feel your mind relaxing. Your face relaxes. Your arms
and your hands ... relax. Your chest and your abdomen
... relax. Your legs and your feet ... relax. *You completely
... relax....*

> Meditation and concentration
> Are the way to a life of serenity.
> Unknown

Yoga Flow

Breathing Exercises

Types of Yoga

Your Yoga Routines

Yoga Flow

Flow happens when your strength, energy, thoughts, and feelings are integrated, moving in the same direction, with the same *intention*, and a focused *attention*, on the same path.

It's a sense of *hooking up*—whether it's your body, your mind, your heart's desires, your day, your entire life, or all of the foregoing. The result of flow is a feeling of being in the right place, doing the right thing, at the right time.

Flow in yoga is a series of physical movements that encourage the practice of flow in your thoughts (mind) and feelings (heart), providing the numerous benefits of stretching, integration, and purpose.

Flow in mind and body reinforces equanimity and a happy, productive, calm, meditative, and peaceful life.

You may each experience your own private flow, and, on occasion, you may discover that you're in a shared, remarkable flow. You can't force it, you can't expect it, but when it happens, it's a gift.

> Hold on to the truth within yourself
> As if it is the only truth.
> Buddha

Pranayama – Yoga Breathing

Yoga and meditation honor being in the moment, and paying attention to your breathing brings you into the moment.

Our bodies are amazing miracles! We breathe and our bodies do all that is connected to the process of breathing, without our having to consciously direct it. What would it be like to have to tell your body to do everything it requires to take a breath?

Breathing generously provides the fuel of life-sustaining oxygen. It relieves tension and stress, calms the nervous system, diminishes fatigue, and reduces high blood pressure with every inhale. It carts off carbon dioxide and toxins with every exhale.

So, when you consciously think about breathing, send gratitude to your body for breathing without being instructed.

Central to yoga practice is conscious attention to the *breath*, altering it so that it activates your parasympathetic nervous system, the "rest and digest" system—the opposite of "fight or flight," where our harried lives hurl us far too often.

"Prana" is your *Life Force*, regulated by your breath. When we breathe consciously, it takes us into a grounded and meditative state. There are a number of

breathing exercises in yoga, let us practice three of the most common ones: *Simha Pranayama* (*Lion's Breath*), *Nadi Shodhana* (*Alternate Nostril Breathing*), and *Ujjayi* (*Ocean Breath*).

Simha Pranayama – Lion's Breath

While practicing *Lion's Breath*, you'll notice that the pranayama cools down your body, and that it also relieves stress and tension.

To practice *Lion's Breath*, breathe deeply through your nose and then quite forcefully exhale through your mouth, with your mouth wide open, tongue sticking out toward your chin, making a '*haaaaaa*' sound. Repeat from 3 to 10 times. Don't be shy—everyone needs to be a lion once in a while!

Nadi Shodhana – Alternate Nostril Breath

Nadi Shodhana comes from two Sanskrit words: *Nadi* = "flow" or "channel," and *Shodhana* = "purification." This breath exercise is focused on clearing the subtle channels of your body, mind, and spirit, while balancing your masculine and feminine energies.

How to Create Nadi Shodhana Breath

Sitting comfortably, keep your back, head, and neck in a straight line. Calmly take three or four deep breaths to become centered. Leave your left hand on your knee. Form the *Vishnu mudra* with your right hand by folding the index and middle fingers to your palm. Alternately, you may place your index and middle fingers between your eyebrows.

Inhale deeply, then with your right thumb, close off your right nostril. Exhale through your left nostril, picturing your breath traveling down the left side of your head, throat, down the left side of your spine through your organs, and down to your pelvic floor. Pause for a moment. Then inhale through your left nostril, picturing your breath traveling up from your pelvic floor up your left side, through all your organs, along the left side of your spine, and up into your throat and head. Pause.

Closing off your left nostril with your ring and pinky fingers, release your right nostril, and exhale, picturing your breath traveling down the right side of your head, throat, down the right side of your spine through your organs, and down to your pelvic floor. Pause. Then inhale through your right nostril, picturing your breath traveling up from your pelvic floor up your right side, through all your organs, along the right side of your spine, and up into your throat and head.

Continue this cycle for 20 or 30 breaths, then complete with an exhalation through your left nostril, and relax your right hand in your lap or on your knee and breath deeply.

A variation is to count on the inhalation up to a comfortable number, for example, six, hold the breath for a count of two, then exhale for a count of six and hold at the bottom of your breath for a count of two. An alternate discipline for this method is to increase the count on the exhale and inhale.

Nadi Shodhana Breath and Your Health

Nadi Shodhana has many benefits. It removes toxins while infusing your body with oxygen. It reduces stress and anxiety. It clears your respiratory channels, and helps to alleviate allergies. It calms and rejuvenates your nervous system.

Nadi Shodhana helps balance your hormones, aids mental clarity, and enhances concentration. It equalizes the right and left hemispheres of your brain, and your masculine-solar, and feminine-lunar, energies.

Ujjayi

"*Ujjayi*" is Sanskrit for "victorious" or "to gain mastery." *Ujjayi* breath sounds like the ocean when it "inhales" coming into shore, and then "exhales," going back out to sea. In fact, this image of the ocean tide coming and going with your breath can help you stay focused on your breathing during your yoga practice.

How to Create Ujjayi Breath

You develop your *Ujjayi* breath by constricting the back of your throat, like when you're about to whisper. *Which you are!* Except you're not going to whisper words, you're going to whisper your breath as you breathe your *Ujjayi* breath through your nose.

Breath in, slowly and deeply, hear the ocean coming into the shore. There's a pause at the top of your breath, and then, slowly release your breath as the wave leaves the shore, returning out to the ocean. Then another pause at the bottom of your breath. Just like the tide, your breath returns again as it flows in and out through your nose.

So relaxing and calming....

Ujjayi Breath with Your Yoga Movements

Here are a few of the reasons why it's good to use *Ujjayi* breath with your yoga movements:

Ujjayi breathing improves concentration during your practice. When you are absorbed in producing your ocean breath, you can remain in poses for longer periods.

Ujjayi breathing releases tension both physically and mentally.

Ujjayi breathing is meditative and deepens the mind-body-spirit connection that is central to yoga. It assists in grounding you and nurtures your self-awareness.

Ujjayi breathing promotes regulated heat for your body. The friction of the air as it passes through your lungs and throat generates internal body heat. This warmed air massages your internal organs, making stretching even more enjoyable, and the positions more readily achieved.

This generated internal heat helps your organs clear out toxins.

Ujjayi Breath and Your Health

You may also discover that *Ujjayi* breath diminishes headaches, relieves sinus pressure and decreases phlegm, all while providing strength for your nervous and digestive systems.

The full, deep, breath of *Ujjayi* breathing helps with the challenges of a yoga practice. As your breathing habit develops, you may discover that it helps with challenges elsewhere in your life as well.

The ancient yogis knew that there's an intimate connection between *breath* and *mind*. Your breath is a teacher. As you learn to pay attention to it, you'll learn much about yourself, encouraging equanimity and strength through all of life's passages.

With practice, you will discover that *Ujjayi*—and all yoga breathing exercises—brings balance into your life on physical, mental, emotional, and spiritual levels.

> When you own your breath,
> Nobody can steal your peace.
> Unknown

Forms of Yoga

There are many forms of yoga, with each their own emphasis. But there are two processes to keep in mind, no matter what form you engage in:

Stay focused on your breath—inhale and exhale through your nose to maintain your body warmth and energy.

Visualize your spine—picture a comfortable space between each vertebra and disk. See, in your mind's eye, each vertebra, each disk, flexible in movement and in stillness, in perfect alignment, balanced and whole.

Many of us have vertebra or disks that are *not* in perfect alignment, that are *not* perfectly whole, but keeping that image in your mind's eye—which is a powerful source of healing, behind *your third eye!*—can contribute to your body's ability to maintain, and to heal.

Following is a short list of the more common forms of yoga:

Hatha Yoga is best for the beginner as it uses a variety of the common poses. It's a classic approach to yoga's poses and breathing exercises.

Iyengar Yoga was founded by B. K. S. Iyengar. It focuses on precise movements, and the details of alignment. Poses are generally held for a long period, while continuing to adjust the fine details of the pose.

Ashtanga Yoga the "Eight Limb path," is a physically demanding sequence of postures, generally more appropriate for the experienced yogi.

Vinyasa Yoga comes from *Ashtanga* as a flowing link of movements, united to the breath. It's not uncommon for a *Vinyasa* flow to be included in *Hatha* Yoga.

Restorative Yoga This book, *Bed Yoga*, takes a restorative approach. *Restorative Yoga* relaxes you, and, as its name implies, it restores you, body and mind and spirit. In this relaxation and restoration, there is also rejuvenation.

No matter what time of day you engage in *Restorative Yoga*, you'll reap the benefit of the three *R's*:
Relaxation
Restoration
Rejuvenation

> Your soul is your best friend
> Treat it with care
> Nurture it with growth
> Feed it with love.
> Ashourina Yalda

Favorite Yoga Routines

One of the many wonderful aspects of yoga is that you can make it yours in any way that suits you best. Here you can write down sequences the two of you have developed that let you completely relax, that empower you, that strengthen your bodies, that enhances your minds, and nurtures your spirits.

A Favorite Restorative Routine:

_____

_____

_____

_____

_____

_____

_____

_____

_____

_____

_____

_____

_____

_____

_____

A Favorite Restorative Routine:

_____

_____

_____

_____

_____

_____

_____

_____

_____

_____

_____

_____

_____

_____

_____

_____

_____

_____

_____

_____

_____

_____

_____

_____

_____

A Favorite Rejuvenating Routine:

_____

_____

_____

_____

_____

_____

_____

_____

_____

_____

_____

_____

_____

_____

_____

_____

_____

_____

_____

_____

_____

_____

_____

A Favorite Rejuvenating Routine:

_____

_____

_____

_____

_____

_____

_____

_____

_____

_____

_____

_____

_____

_____

_____

_____

_____

_____

_____

_____

_____

_____

_____

_____

_____

Your Gift ....

Here's the link to your free copy of
Save Your Life with Stupendous Spices
as a thank you for purchasing *Bed Yoga for Couples*:

https://BookHip.com/DKHVDA

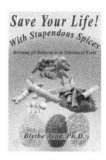

Or you may write to me for your copy:
Blythe@BlytheAyne.com

About the Author

I live in a forest with a few domestic and numerous wild creatures, where I create an ever-growing inventory of books, both nonfiction and fiction, short stories, illustrated kid's books, and articles, with a bit of wood carving when I need a change of pace.

I've practiced yoga for decades with amazing teachers, always keeping for myself a beginner, no competition, mindset.

I received my Doctorate from the University of California at Irvine in the School of Social Sciences, majoring in psychology and ethnography, after which I moved to the Pacific Northwest to write and to have a modest private psychotherapy practice in a small town not much bigger than a village. Finally I decided it was time to put my full focus on my writing, where, through the world-shrinking internet, I could "meet" greater numbers of people. *Where I could meet you!*

All the creatures in my forest and I thank you for "stopping by" and sharing some quiet, healing yoga. If **Bed Yoga for Couples** has touched you in a positive way I hope you'll consider writing a review, as reviews are an author's life blood, and are an excellent means for other people to discover books that might inspire them on their way.

I Wish You Happiness, Health, Peace, and Joy,
Blythe

Questions, comments? I'd love to hear from you!:

Blythe@BlytheAyne.com

www.BlytheAyne.com

Printed in Great Britain
by Amazon

76066834R00068